THE SECRET INGREDIENT

HOW TO UNLOCK WEIGHT
LOSS THAT LASTS FOR LIFE

———————————————

Marie Ann Mosher, CPT, AADP,CHHC

Beyond Food Publishing

ISBN: 978-0692313817

Printed in USA

Dedication

This book is dedicated to Natasia Lotte,
who always remembers to add
The Secret Ingredient !

Contents

How to Use This Book

I challenge you to read this book in its entirety. It is not necessary to believe or use everything in this book. Grab hold of the concepts you find useful and put them into action immediately! You will not have to implement all the action items and strategies in this book to transform the quality of your life. All the strategies and techniques have individual potential to change your life. When used together, however, they will produce amazing results that will stay with you for life.

I hope this will be a book you will read again and again. The purpose is to take your life to a whole new level. Please consider this book an indispensable tool in creating health for life.

Preface

All my life, I have taken incredible pleasure in making and enjoying delicious food.

As a teenager, I had already begun experimenting and creating my own recipes. I loved food and everything about it! It wasn't long before that I rarely used a recipe or cracked open a cookbook unless it was to look for an idea about a general concept. Most often, I came up with ideas on my own and proceeded to do what felt right.

I knew before I even finished high school that I wanted to major in Nutritional Science in college so I could understand exactly how foods nourish our bodies and how to make them taste even better.

After completing my bachelor's degree, I worked as a food scientist for several years and even went on to open my own restaurant. Yet, I still hungered for a better understanding of true nutrition. I decided to attend a holistic nutrition school, the Institute for Integrative Nutrition, hoping to understand the connection between feeding our bodies and nourishing our souls.

For years, though, I continued stuffing my face with every "healthy" food imaginable. I ate raw, vegan, organic and local foods. You name it….. I ate it! I still felt hungry, though. As though something HUGE was missing. So, I used volumetrics, a strategy focused on eating a large volume of food but with minimal calories, to stuff loads of food into my body hoping to ease the hunger in my soul and fill my body with the right nutrients. I understood the physical act of supplying nutrients but the soul filling aspect of nourishment was missing.

After years of these antics, my energy was low, my hair was falling out, my anxiety levels were high and I was just plain unhappy. I couldn't understand it. I was eating the right things. But, somehow they weren't "working". I was ultimately shocked when I found out my health was seriously declining despite my best efforts.

It took some soul searching and realizing the implications of my diminishing health to see that I had been missing the most vital ingredient for quite sometime. I realized - love, energy, intention and gratitude….the components that comprise the Secret Ingredient had eluded me where it mattered most. For so much of my life, I had been transferring fear, guilt and anxiety to my food and making things worse instead of better.

Somehow, I had thought the nutrients would overpower the dis-ease within my life. It took sometime but I learned how to slow down, to give myself the love and nourishment I needed without looking to food as the only way to fill my soul. I began experimenting with what foods truly spoke to me instead of just eating those that were statistically best. Investigating where the most calming and centering places were for me to eat.

I considered when I should eat. I starting becoming comfortable with the fact that my best time to eat might not coincide with other people's optimal mealtime.

I started making the act of food preparation one of love and passion. I relearned how to eat. Throwing the notion of utensils out the window, I transferred my energy and love through my own hands. I savored each morsel with gusto. I became mindful while eating, explored my gratitude towards the food itself and everything involved it how it came to me.

I also began learning the importance of my time spent after eating and how to continue the gratitude and assimilation of love and energy through the digestion process with long walks and mindfulness.

It was only natural when my daughter came along, that she and I began creating recipes together. When we would make our recipes, we would continually taste and perfect them. At the end, I would ask my daughter if it was ready yet or if we needed to add anything else. Finally, she would say that it was perfect. Then, I would teasingly ask, "Have you added the secret ingredient yet?"

We would both giggle and clasp our hands tightly over our hearts. Then, we would express gratitude for the food before us, give our intention for the meal to nourish us and convey love to everyone who would eat it. Last, we would open our hands and gently sprinkle the secret ingredient into the bowl.

One day while my daughter was still a preschooler, we had been talking for days about making our own special version of yogurt in our blender. When we finally decided to make the yogurt and had finished adding all the ingredients, I asked Natasia if we all set to blend. My daughter said, "wait mommy, you forgot to add the secret ingredient".

Teasingly, I asked Natasia what the secret ingredient was and she shouted, "Love mommy, it's the love!" Then, she held up a beautiful picture she had drawn. It was an image of her mixing all the ingredients including an abundance of hearts to signify the love.

I'll never forget how proud I was when I realized Natasia knew the importance of love, energy, intention and gratitude at such a young age. From that day forward, we have always made a point to put the secret ingredient into our food and help others do the same.

With Love and Gratitude
Marie Ann Mosher

Introduction

Have you ever tasted a meal so truly wonderful that you felt compelled to ask what made the recipe so special? Were you told, "It's my secret ingredient!"?

Have you ever considered that the secret ingredient may not actually be a physical tangible component of the recipe but and actual energy or force emanating from the cook themselves?

Could it be possible that intentions and energy vibrations make the difference in how the food tastes and how well it nourishes us?

If you knew that electromagnetic power of the heart is 5,000 times stronger than that of the brain, would you consider this notion?

Imagine a world where it's not about what you buy. It's about what you put forth from inside you. Imagine an equal playing field, where we all have the same opportunity to put nourishment into our lives and body. This nourishment is the energy and vibration that comes from love.

Have you ever wondered how a person with access to the best foods could have poor physical health? And yet a person with access to just enough food to survive is thriving and flourishing?

The difference is gratitude, intention and love versus apathy, disdain and disregard. According to the research done by Massaru Emoto for his book "Messages in Water", the only emotion with higher vibrational energy than love is GRATITUDE!

In The Secret Ingredient you will be guided in how to select your food with love and intention. Then, supported in determining where the optimal place is for you, personally, to eat. Then, mentored in deciding when the optimal time each day is for you to eat. You will also learn how to prepare foods using your very own "Secret Ingredient" to deliver maximum energy and nourishment to yourself and those you make meals for.

Next, you will be guided in creating an optimal eating environment or making the most of the environment available to you. Then you will be taken on a journey of learning how to eat again. Eating with gratitude, love and acceptance.

The secret ingredient also tackles the vital issue of "when not to eat". Putting yourself first and realizing that eating at a designated time, location or when others are ready may not be best for you, personally.

You will be introduced to the notion that what happens after you eat is also as important as the act of eating itself.

Last, the secret ingredient will provide you vital tools to optimize your eating experience and show you that your thoughts are nourishment as well as the physical "food" you consume!

Chapter 1
Top Secret

" If you want to find the secrets of the universe think in terms of energy, frequency and vibration "- Nikola Tesla

What exactly is the secret ingredient?

Why is it so important?

Have you spent countless hours searching for the perfect diet?

Or on the never-ending quest for the perfect foods?

Looking for the proverbial "Secret Ingredient" for health, energy, weight loss and vitality?

Within: A Spiritual Awakening to Love & Weight Loss, written Dr. Habib Sadeghi sums up the answer quite concisely and elegantly in the following excerpt:

It was in a conference at the University of Southern California in 1995 that physicist Edward Witten of the Institute for Advanced Study stunned the world when he presented his M-Theory. Building upon the work of physicist Leonard Susskind of Stanford University in the 1970s, Witten's M-Theory or String Theory was both shocking and beautiful. It said that physical matter isn't truly real. Everything, whether it's a tree, a butterfly, or your body is all made up of exactly the same thing: infinitesimally small vibrating strands of energy.

What makes them appear in different forms is simply the rate or frequency at which those strands are vibrating. Not only was this discovery a boon for science, but also it gave credence to the mystics and sages who have said for millennia that we are all ONE and that everything is the same thing. THOUGHTS BECOME THINGS.

So if everything is just energy in vibration, what controls the rate of that vibration to make you, you? The answer is: your thoughts. Thought waves have their own frequency much like gamma waves, radio waves, or microwaves, and they are the conductors that mold the very energy that makes up (Sadeghi, 2014).

Sadeghi, H. (2014). *Within: A Spiritual Awakening to Love & Weight Loss*. Los Angeles, California: Premier Digital Publishing.

The principles of quantum physics also provide information that relates directly to health and healing. Since our bodies are made of carbon, hydrogen, oxygen, nitrogen and minerals that are found throughout the universe, it means that these components are part of plants, animals, water, air, etc and are recycled many times.

The components that make up these elements are protons, neutrons and electrons, which can be traced directly to vibrations and energy. Therefore, the body can be understood in terms of energy.

Thus, there are infinite possibilities for change when an entity is compromised of energy. Therefore, we are not stuck with the current challenges, ailments, etc in our bodies. There are infinite possibilities and opportunities for change. In the quantum realm nothing is fixed, there are vast possibilities.

What used to be an apple becomes part of your body and what used to be part of you becomes part of the leaf of a plant as you breathe out the carbon and oxygen in the form of carbon dioxide.

Nothing is constant in your body. It is continually changing all the time. If your body is experiencing illness, it is also possible to experience wellness.

You must take responsibility to step towards wellness.

"In the quantum realm everything is interwoven and inseparably one" (Sadeghi, 2014). When you eat or drink something, those atoms and molecules become part of you and your body.

Intention creates reality. Thus, is illness a blessing or a curse? Awareness gives you power and control over your life.

Hippocrates said, "For this is the great error of our day: that the physicians separate the soul from the body". The body and soul are one system. The mind is in the body.

Are you aware that there is actuallya neuropeptide in the body that specifically carries emotionally charged memories and information that is imbedded through the body? Thus, we each possess a network of these molecules that create our feelings and beliefs. This is why "The body follows what is in the heart and mind of the person".

Human beings are wired for wholeness and happiness. It is different for each of us. **The answer is inside you.**

LOVE

According to Bruce Lipton, 90% of people don't LOVE themselves! Cell Biologist Bruce Lipton spent his career investigating positive thinking and how it powers the cells of our system to fight disease and regenerate the body.

According to Lipton, "the brain controls the behavior of the body's cells" and that "harnessing the power of your mind can be more effective than the drugs you have been programmed to believe you need".

Consider this: have you ever eaten a meal made by your grandma that tasted so good, every bite was like heaven? I bet, you begged for the recipe. Then, when you made it, things never quite tasted the same?

What was it that was so different, when your grandma made the recipe?

She used the Secret Ingredient. Love. Energy. Gratitude. Your grandma put herself into the food.

My whole life, I have spent hours in the kitchen preparing even some of the simplest meals. I've been asked "Why can't you just take a piece of bread, slap a slice of cheese on it and eat it, like everyone else ?" Hmmn. Well, I'd never actually thought of that. To me preparing food is like creating art. I love devising meals that are incredibly appealing to the eyes, meals that are so

---

beautiful you are almost were afraid to eat them. Yet, your mouth waters so much, you know that you have to!

Many people have asked me that same question during my life. Yet to me, I think, how could you possibly eat food that is not beautiful? I have always taken great care just to arrange a meal just so. To put care into the shape of the cuts of vegetables.

For years, people have been telling me my food preparations look so good, like they weren't even real. Like artwork. That they were afraid to eat it because it looks so good. I always thought this strange. Wouldn't you want to eat food that looks like artwork?

I have also, always, taken care to make even the simplest salad vivid and eye catching. Wouldn't that be all the more reason to eat it? To enjoy the love and care I took to put my heart, energy and self into the food?

People have always asked me why my salads and sandwiches taste better than anything they've ever eat. To that I always smile and say, "It's my secret ingredient".

WATER

Let's also take note that Masaru Emoto, the author of *Messages in Water*, researched water extensively and that food is primarily water. Emoto determined that water is actually affected by our energy and vibration. Considering that our bodies are 70% water this is quite significant. If water can be influenced by our thoughts and energy, no wonder a bad mood can have such impact on our physiology!

(NOTE: Ideally, it is best to use spring water or well water. Water that has been chlorinated will not have the same energy or transfer positive energy the way fresh water will.)

The traditional theories of old biology taught that we were victims of our heredity. Now, we know that cells are affected greatly by environment NOT just heredity !

Nikola Tessla said "EVERYTHING IS ENERGY" and he was right. Even Albert Einstein realized the energy potential of food!

So, What is the Secret Ingredient?

You, your love, gratitude and energy.

Why is it important ??

Health
Longevity
Happiness
Vitality

It was Nobel Prize-winning quantum physicist Werner Heisenberg who said, "Atoms or elementary particles themselves are not real; they form a world of potentialities or possibilities rather than one of things or facts."

The way food is grown, harvested, prepared and eaten emotionally charges the food. Likewise, taste and smell aren't the only senses that emotionally charge food. All five senses contribute to the charge our food holds to us.

Eating combines the intelligence of humanity and nature. Our senses are the pathways that comingle this intelligence. Ideally, food would be grown with consciousness, kind harvest, and mindful preparation then eaten with intention, mindfulness and true presence. Mindfulness directs and connects our actions from a state of peace and calm.

When eating foods without this love and intention, bodies try to replicate a natural feeling of peace and calm by attaching to certain food. This is the root of emotional eating. We must embed our food and lives with love and intention to break this mental connection of food with peace and calm. This, can take time to overcome because of the "sensory stimulation" that emotionally charged foods give.

CHANGE

Again referencing the eloquent words of Dr. Habib Sadeghi, we realize that:

The only thing constant is the ever-flowing energy that we all reside in that's forever changing form based on the rate of vibration it takes on. Everything in life is built on a continuous cycle of regeneration and renewal.

Winter always turns to spring. The moon gives way to the sun each morning. Earth that was charred and barren from wildfires soon sprouts green with life again. While it may look the same to you year to year, even your body is in a constant state of renewal. Everyone knows hair, skin and fingernail cells continue to grow throughout life.

What science is finally discovering is that virtually every cell in your body is renewed on a regular basis. This includes cells for organs for which regeneration was once thought impossible, such as the brain and heart.

A study recently performed at the Karolinska Institute in Stockholm, Sweden, has proven that human beings actually regenerate heart cells throughout their entire life span. Radioactive isotope studies are showing that you get a new stomach lining every five years (Sadeghi, 2014)

Don't look for things outside yourself to fill voids in your life.

Everything you need, you already have and everything you want, you already are. Access that place inside yourself where all things are possible.

We are all connected. Thus, it is impossible for you to be alone. It is also impossible for someone else to better than you because we are all part of each other and interconnected.

Nothing outside of you will ever fulfill you. Therefore, you must look inside yourself to find the secret ingredient.

We know now that only emotion with higher vibrational energy than love is gratitude. So, we must be thankful for every morsel of food in your life and every drop of liquid. Each bite contributes to who you are and who you will be in the future.

So, start today. This is not something to put off until a time when you are less busy or stressed!

Everything we feed ourselves now builds the foundation for which we become.

Don't feed yourself will hurry, frenzy and worry.

Feed yourself with love, calm and acceptance.

Chapter 2

This, That and the Other Thing
What To Eat

"Every 35 days, your skin replaces itself and your body makes new cells from the food you eat. What you eat literally becomes you"

What do you eat?

Do you eat fast food?

Processed food?

Do you eat foods that truly nourish you?

Do you feel good when you eat it?

If you've just been eating whatever is convenient, it may be time to step back and consider how this choice is affecting your health.

Eat only the foods You WANT to EAT

This may be the first time in your life anyone has every told you this but here goes: ONLY eat what you WANT to eat. Never eat what you think you should eat or someone else tells you must eat.

How can you truly enjoy your meal, if it has been forced upon you?

What to eat? Start by finding foods that speak to you. Look. Touch. Feel. Smell. Choose Foods that resonate with you. It doesn't matter what other people think. Your body will actually tell you what you need! Your body is very wise. You may be craving a specific nutrient. It's okay to eat zucchini for three days, if that's what your body (you) is saying it needs.

If you craving things that aren't really **FOOD**, then take a look deeper and figure out what emotion is causing the craving or what emotional nourishment you are trying to receive through the food.

When eating foods without love and intention our bodies try to replicate a natural feeling of peace and calm by attaching to certain food. This is the root of emotional eating. We must embed our food and lives with love and intention to break this mental connection of food with peace and calm.

This can take time to overcome because of the "sensory stimulation" that emotionally charged foods give off. We can smell trillions of different scents. Just the scent of food can carry emotionally charged feelings and memories. This can trigger a cascade of memories and an ingrained psychological response. It can even determine whether or not you like the food, independent of the actual taste.

So, throw the advice out the window of making it a must to eat Brussels sprouts, broccoli, etc. If you have a bad memory from childhood you are doing yourself more harm than good but eating those things.

Likewise, if you have a positive memory associated with a certain food it will affect how you feel about it. I associate turkey grinders as a comforting experience of love and support because I used to eat them when I was with my dad. This is not what I would consider the healthiest meal but it is nourishing to me because of the positive associations.

REAL Food

"Eat food. Not too much. Mostly plants."

For all the millions of pages written about eating well, these seven words sum it up best. This quote from Michael Pollan, the author of *The Omnivore's Dilemma*, captures the essence of what we need to know to enjoy a long, healthy life.

"Eat food." By this, he means REAL food. The kind of food that comes from nature, that grows in the ground or on trees or on the ocean floor. Food that comes from animals who are treated well and not poisoned with chemicals or whose products come to us tainted by how they are raised, slaughtered, and processed. This is the kind of food that will go bad if you don't eat it within a few days, because it's not been fortified with artificial preservatives intended to ensure a long shelf life (and as few nutrients as possible).

Remember this helpful adage: the longer the shelf life of a food you eat, the shorter YOUR shelf life will be. If you can't pronounce the ingredients on a food label without a chemistry degree, then it is NOT healthy!

"Mostly plants." Certainly, some people find nourishment, comfort, and strength from animal products like meat, fish, and dairy. But most of us eat far more of these kinds of foods than our bodies can possibly process and properly digest.

And many of us cannot only live without them, but we thrive when we replace them with plant-based foods. When we eat high nutrient foods, we find that not only are our bellies full and satisfied, but we feel their effects throughout our bodies – and beyond.

So, how can we begin to put Pollan's simple little philosophy into practice? Here are the principles that, generally speaking, apply to all of us.

Start with greens

Greens, greens, and lots of them! Greens are the most nutrient dense foods on the planet. The darker, the better. Eating salads helps ensure you get a lot of your greens raw. When cooking, steam them briefly – or you can even bake them on a low heat in the oven for a crispy chip-like texture.

Why Greens?

Foods like spinach, kale, collards, swiss chard, bok choy, watercress, parsley, mustard greens, turnip greens – these are the foods with the most nutrients in the purest form, with the fewest amount of calories per serving.

As we know, Americans eat fewer leafy green vegetables than any other food. We need them the most, but eat them the least, and our waistlines are proof.

Add a wide variety of vegetables to your meals.

There are so many options in the produce department, so here's a chance to experiment with new flavors. Eggplants, squash, zucchini, carrots, sweet potatoes, onions, mushrooms, cucumbers, radishes... the list goes on and on.

If you are unaccustomed to eating vegetables, it might take a little while to get your palate adjusted to their tastes and textures. But the key to getting all the various vitamins and nutrients available is color. A variety of colors every day will ensure a good mix of different nutrients to fuel your body exceptionally well.

Make sure your body is hydrated.

This means hydrated with water, not DEhydrated by coffee, soda, beer, or other drinks. Conventional wisdom says 64 ounces a day is an ideal amount. But you need to let your body dictate how much water consumption is optimal for you.

Lots of greens, lots of vegetables, and adequate water – are the most universally applicable rules. The following are generally applicable:

Fruits: Most of us should eat a serving or two of fruit a day. Foods like berries provide a huge dose of antioxidants. Apples are a good source of fiber, bananas give us potassium, avocados have healthy fats… every fruit has several benefits, in fact. A word of caution, however, for people with diabetes or other blood sugar issues: Most fruits do contain fructose, and this can be problematic in the diets of some people. Though the sugar is natural, sugar is sugar. It can lead to weight gain or other more serious complications, so leaning more toward low fructose fruits are your best bet. And moderation is key.

Whole grains: Whole grains are the unprocessed kind, not the highly refined and "enriched" products we see in the bags of white sandwich bread and boxes of "instant" white rice on the supermarket shelves. "Refined" and "enriched" sound like such positive words, but don't be fooled. Refined grain has been stripped of its raw nutrients and does little more than spike your blood sugar through its empty calories. It tends to be "white" food, or sometimes colored with an artificial ingredient to cover up its "whiteness," as in the case with many so-called "wheat" breads.

A good rule of thumb is to avoid foods such as white rice, white breads, pastas and even possibly white potatoes. Try red or sweet potatoes for a change, brown rice instead of white, and be adventurous with other grains as well – it's not hard to find tasty recipes that call for quinoa, millet, and barley. Truly whole grain breads have very few ingredients besides the grains and whole wheat flour. You can even find live sprouted grain breads that don't have flour, which are excellent sources of protein and fiber.

Beans and legumes: These nutrient powerhouses are tremendously high in protein and fiber. If you aren't used to eating them, you may experience a bit of digestive discomfort at first. But as your overall diet improves over time, that tends to ease up. There are endless varieties of soups, casseroles, dips and Mexican dishes you can prepare starting with beans.

Nuts and Seeds: Avoid the roasted, salted, and oiled kinds. And of course, if you're allergic, avoid them in all forms. But for the rest of us, raw nuts and seeds, as well as nut and seed butters, are excellent sources of protein and nutrients, and they also aid in the absorption of nutrients from greens in smoothies and salads.

Nuts in particular are high in calories and should be enjoyed in moderation – a handful is an adequate serving for most of us.

A diet of greens, vegetables, fruits, whole grains, beans, legumes, nuts and seeds – along with adequate water intake – is a fantastic foundation for our overall eating plan. With very few exceptions, a diet consisting of just these foods can get our weight quickly under control, prevent all our modern lifestyle diseases, and even reverse them in people who already have them. Many people – former President Bill Clinton is perhaps the most famous example – stick to this way of eating and have no desire or need to consume anything else, while protecting themselves from cancer, heart attacks, diabetes, and a whole host of other health concerns.

But, while consuming more of these foods is a health benefit to almost everyone, eating only these foods doesn't work for everyone. In the next chapter, we'll have some suggestions for figuring out how to develop an individualized eating plan that works specifically for YOU.

SNACKING

1.   **Nuts and Seeds**. These are the best and most convenient all natural snacks you can keep around. Unlike fruits and vegetables, they keep for some time. You can buy them in bulk and not worry about running to the store every few days to replenish them. Stock up on raw, unsalted varieties you like. Almonds and walnuts have tremendous health benefits, as do sunflower and sesame seeds.

If you are watching your weight, stick to just a handful a day, as the natural fats, although healthy, can work against a plan to lose weight. Slivered almonds might be preferable to the whole kind in this instance. Quite often I mix a handful of nuts and seeds with raisins, which makes for a very satisfying and healthy protein rich snack with a variety of tastes in a small portion.

2.   **Veggie trays and dips**. Vegetables actually make fantastic snacks, even more so when paired with a tasty dip. Carrots, celery, cucumbers and broccoli might be a bit challenging to get into your blender, but you can find them conveniently cut and packaged in the produce section of almost any grocery store. They also tend to be paired in those packages with a dip that is based in a processed, high fat ranch dressing, which isn't exactly optimal for health.

So, I recommend you find a nice hummus dip to complement this snack. Made from garbanzo beans, it's a delicious way to spice up the vegetables that might be lacking the flavors your taste buds are used to. They make all kinds of hummus these days, too – with garlic, pine nuts, lemon, roasted peppers, you name it.

You can find other healthy dips if hummus isn't your thing or you want to mix things up – there are some great bean dips (not the refried kind!), delicious guacamole and all natural salsas ranging from mild to super hot. If you're inclined, of course you could make all these dips yourself. But if you're pressed for time and want the "convenience" factor, you can find all these foods prepared and packaged without preservatives or artificial ingredients. Read the ingredient labels and purchase something that clearly shows only whole foods in the list.

4.   **Five apples and five bananas.** These traditional, common fruits are easy to bring, eat, and dispose of. No need for a knife to peel. Take your time and pick out the best looking apples you can find – and if you like and don't mind peeling, find some other fruits, too.

Set up a bowl on your desk to store them. The attractive arrangement will also brighten your mood the way a fresh bouquet of flowers or a sturdy plant would.

5.   **Whole food bars.** There have been lots of energy and meal replacement bars on the market for decades now. The problem with most of them is that they are highly processed and laden with sugar and high fructose corn syrup. They won't help your health goals any more than a Snickers bar would.

Brands such as Larabar, Pure Bar, and Amazing Greens (to name a few) have developed the technology to produce whole food bars without any of those artificial or sugary ingredients. Lots of these bars come in chocolate varieties, flavored with nutrient rich cacao and sweetened with dried fruit. Again, read labels religiously.

And if you want to make your own, here's a ridiculously simple recipe for raw vegan brownies that will take as long to make as it does for you to get from the power bar section in your grocery store, through the checkout, and into your car!

1 cup of pitted mejool dates
1 cup of walnuts
¼ cup of cacao powder

Blend all of the above in a blender or food processor and press into a small baking dish. Refrigerate or freeze. Makes nine small but very filling brownies.

Another sweet treat? Take the above ingredients and after blending, instead of pressing into a pan, crumble and sprinkle over fresh raspberries. Decadently healthy!

6.   **All natural chips and crackers.** Sometimes, we do crave a little salt and a little crunch. If you can handle eating them in moderation, look in the snack section for products that are few in ingredients, and whose ingredients begin with whole grains. There are certain crackers, tortilla and rice chips on the market that fit the bill and also pair nicely with the aforementioned salsas and hummus dips.

Better yet, try to make some crunchy, salty things on your own, like kale chips! Just remove the leaves from the stems, coat them with a little grapeseed oil, bake for five to ten minutes at 350 degrees, then sprinkle with some sea salt as soon as you remove them. Delicious!

Try to make an effort to drink your smoothies and eat these snacks before you indulge in any other foods around the office, especially when special occasions pop up to sabotage your efforts to eat better.

Don't skip the foods on holidays or other treats you might like if you want them. But you may just find that with a smoothie or two, a handful of carrots, and that spectacular peanut butter and jelly sandwich in your system, those other foods don't appeal to you quite the way they did before. Amazing what real food can do!

No more processed or manufactured junk!

Did you know that Every 35 days, your skin replaces itself and your body makes new cells from the food you eat? What you eat literally becomes you. So, please, eat foods REAL foods.

If you are short on time prepare a mono meal and put your heart into it. A mono meal is an entire meal comprised of one type of food. For example, all beans or all broccoli. This makes digestion easier on your system and makes preparation quick and easy. Depending on the item you choose there may be no preparation at all.

If preparation is required, making something amazing can take 5 minutes but is so much better than rushing for 20 minutes and putting that horrible energy into your food. Choose to Consume foods that are easy to digest - cucumbers, sprouts and foods with high water content.

Foods with higher water content will give your body higher vibrational energy. Foods with low water content can actually pull water from your body. This is why it's important to eat foods that are as fresh as possible or to grow your own.

The options I like to keep handy are:

Fresh cut organic green beans
Romaine lettuce
Carrots
Sweet peppers
Cut cucumbers
Almonds
Green apples and red apples
Olives
Sugar snap peas
Jicama
Baby spinach
Celery
Pumpkin seeds

And always start with sprouts as the base for any meal!

HYDRATION

Americans are notorious for walking around the office with the ubiquitous cup of coffee in the mornings, often with cream and sugar. And many follow in the afternoons with soda to keep going – high test or the diet kind, either kind of soft drink is again filled with additives, preservatives, high fructose corn syrup or artificial sweeteners proven to cause cancer in rats and suspected to do the same in humans.

As bad as the sugar, cream, and aspartame can be, the caffeine itself is addictive and suspected of contributing to a whole host of health concerns. Of course, there are studies that also point to some possible health benefits of caffeine and coffee, so the data really is inconclusive. But any potential benefits of caffeine come from moderate consumption, not addiction.

In any case, virtually every American walks through his or her day in a state of dehydration. We simply don't drink enough of the one and only drink Mother Nature provides us completely free of charge: water.

The standard recommendation of eight 8 ounce glasses a day doesn't exactly apply to everyone; we all have varying levels of need for water, and it takes a while to figure out what works for each of us.

If you take the time to work through how and what you drink during the day, you'll probably be surprised by the difference you'll feel in no time.

1.   **Water**. Add one full glass of water to your day, preferably early in the morning. In fact, if you are able to consume 16 ounces in the morning on an empty stomach, you'll get the incomparable benefit of a daily early morning detox. And you'll notice a difference as early as day one!

Perhaps you can bring a big bottle to sit on your desk and sip it throughout the day, or find another means of H2O delivery that works for you. But if you aren't drinking enough, don't start out trying to drink a gallon at once. It won't work. Try one glass a day, and see how it feels to you.

2.   **Coffee and Tea**. If you are a coffee addict, or even if you stick to one or two cups a day, try a cup of tea this morning. Flavor it however you like – preferably naturally! – but experiment with something other than just coffee beans: chai tea, green tea, white tea, or any of the dozens of herbal teas on the market.

Many kinds of teas are much lower in caffeine and high in antioxidants. Some are also known to calm the nerves, which is often the exact opposite of the effect that coffee has.

3.   **Soda**. There are different reasons why people drink soda. It would be a good idea for you to take some time to examine what your reasons are. It might be that it's a convenient option in a nearby vending machine. If that's the case, again it goes back to planning ahead to make provisions for yourself.

If it's the "fizz factor," there are lots of carbonated drinks that can fit the bill, without all the unhealthy side effects. Try simple sparkling mineral water, or a version flavored with lemon, lime, or raspberries. (All natural, of course! No sugar, syrup, or aspartame!)

If you really want a sweet taste, try this half and half recipe: fill your glass halfway with sparkling water, and halfway with your favorite all natural fruit juice.

There is also a soda on the market that effectively uses Stevia, an all-natural plant sweetener, to produce a remarkably sweet soda that you might enjoy if you're just not ready to kick the habit. If you drink soda, try drinking one of these alternatives in the afternoon at a time when you'd ordinarily grab that Coke or diet Pepsi. And if you like, experiment with all the options until you find the one that works the best for you.

Notice this plan doesn't call for you to give up your coffee, soda, or sweet tea. Just add these three drinks to your day – one glass of water, one cup of tea, and one sparkling drink. Give it some time to see how these might become new habits you'll want to keep. And maybe after a while, you'll even find you won't want to hang on to the old ones.

YOU ARE UNIQUE

Now that we know the basic foods everyone should eat, how do we figure out the rest? If we each have a different body that needs different foods in different amounts, how can we know exactly what to do?

Well, one thing NOT to do is to buy just any book on healthful eating and follow it religiously. Have you ever noticed how many diet and healthy eating books are on the shelves of your local bookstore? It's overwhelming, and new books, studies, and programs are developed all the time. Each one claims to have the cure to losing weight / staying young / building muscle / gaining energy in its pages. Give up carbs, restrict calories, eat low fat, eat high fat, cut out sugar, eat at certain times, eat this but not that, go vegan, go raw, load up on protein. You can eat for your blood type, rate every food you eat on the glycemic index, try the Atkins plan, cure your belly fat, or eat to address hormonal imbalances.

Every theory is backed up by some kind of empirical evidence, years of research and trials and proof that they work.

The truth is, if any one of these plans had THE answer to achieving optimum health for everyone, it would be the ONLY plan.

All these books have made it on the shelves of the bookstores for two reasons. One, because each one of these plans HAS worked for SOMEONE. And two, because the rest of us are looking for the plan that will work for US.

You can certainly read all those books, and the odds are good one of them will provide the basic elements of an eating style you can live with - and maybe even thrive with - for the rest of your life. But how will you know which diet is right for you?

To start with, you won't. It will take time, patience, and a willingness to experiment with foods you love while determining which ones also love you back. Also remember – don't eat foods that you are allergic to or intolerant of. And if something makes you feel bad, don't eat it! Keep journaling and working this out for yourself, and in time, you'll have written your own diet book – the one that applies just to you.

As noted in the previous chapter, a few basics apply. Whole foods, mostly plants, eaten in great abundance, are the best weapons to prevent and even reverse disease as well as upgrade the quality of your life.

Beyond that, it's up to each of us to figure out what works in other food groups. Some people can figure this out on their own, but it requires patience and experimentation. Just as there are several ways of eating, there are several ways of beginning to determine the best way of eating for you:

---

1.   Crowding out. Instead of eliminating things from your diet, make a conscious effort to incorporate more good things. If you don't usually eat salads, you could add one to your lunch every day. Try the green smoothies, and resolve to drink at least one serving a day. Add in a handful of carrots, change from salted mixed nuts to raw almonds and walnuts, eat an apple in the afternoons, drink an extra glass of water a day – these are just a few examples of ways you can add healthy habits into your routine. Add enough of them in, and you'll have no choice but to crowd out the less healthy choices.

2.   Gradually eliminate things from your diet based on bad habits you want to conquer or ailments from which you are suffering. For instance, if you feel sluggish, you might want to try eliminating dairy from your diet for a week.

        If you haven't been eating breakfast and want to figure out what will best get your motor going in the mornings, spend a week trying different foods for breakfast, and making notes about the effects they have on your energy, digestion, and sense of mental clarity.

Some people thrive on green smoothies, others prefer the grounding properties of a warm bowl of rolled oats with fruit. Still others find the protein in fresh eggs to be an essential staple in a healthy morning breakfast.

3.   Do a whole foods detox, then experiment by adding things back in. If you have the discipline and determination to spend at least five days detoxing your body with a whole foods, plant-based, smoothie and/or juice detox, your body will be more aware of how other foods affect it. Be sure to add other foods in one at a time, so you know what food is having what kind of effect on you. Reintroduce dairy one week, meat the next. You may even find after detoxing that you no longer have a taste for certain foods you used to crave.

No matter what style of eating works for you, the main premise is that a high nutrient diet is critical.

Try this one day sample menu intended to get flavorful, super nutrient dense foods into your diet. Again, you might not find that you enjoy all these foods, or your body might not tolerate them. But until you try and experiment, you won't know.

- *Breakfast:* Large green smoothie, raw almond butter with all natural fruit jam on sprouted grain toast, herbal tea
- *Lunch:* Small green smoothie or pure vegetable juice, huge salad with your favorite veggies, fruits, nuts and greens, balsamic vinaigrette dressing,
- *Snack:* Handful of walnuts with raisins
- *Dinner:* Mexican vegetable and bean soup flavored with cilantro, whole grain tortillas with salsa and black beans
- *Dessert:* strawberry-chocolate smoothie – recipe below:

¼ cup coconut milk, ¼ cup pure water, 5 dates, pitted and soaked in the water, ¼ avocado, 1 cup of fresh spinach, 1 tablespoon of raw cacao, ¼ cup frozen strawberries

Pour the milk and water into the blender with the dates, avocado, and cacao on top. Blend. Add the spinach and strawberries and blend until completely smooth. Serves 1-2.

NATURAL STATE

Try to choose foods in their natural state. It might seem amazing that you can transform food into so many things through baking, frying, pulverizing but just try eating foods exactly as they are.

Pick up a delicious sweet red pepper, take a bite and just chew. **This is nature at its finest!** Heating foods can decrease the vibrational energy, destroy vital nutrients and denature the proteins. This is why I suggest that you aim for 60 - 80 % of your intake as raw fruits, vegetables, nuts and seeds.

Did you know twice the protein is absorbed from raw food as opposed to cooked food? So you can actually eat less raw food and be more nourished while maintaining an optimal weight and health!

CHOOSE LOCAL

Please, choose foods that are local when possible. Yes, I know this seems like some new uppity way of doing things but before the massive advances in transportation, people only ate local. Plus, the truth is that if you eat local foods, the nutrient levels are highest and you are getting the most bang for your buck with every bite!

When picking out the vegetables at the store, look at them lovingly. Go to a farmers and choose the fruits and vegetables that stand out to you. They don't need to be the most beautiful or biggest. Actually the best tasting foods can be small, odd shaped or even scarred. If purchasing from a Community Supported Agriculture Program - opt to help out and get your hands in the soil.

Did you know that if we plant seeds ourselves that they adapt to our individual nutritional needs?

According to Bruce Lipton, this transfer occurs through interspecies gene sharing. Thus, planting your own garden is vital! Even if it is just a kitchen windowsill garden comprised of micro-greens!

OPTIONS

If you are too busy to grow the plants yourself try to get to know the farmer. Take your time and peruse a farmers market. Choosing the fruits and vegetables that appeal to you.

Lipton, B. (2008). *The Biology of Belief: Unleashing the Power of Consciousness, Matter and Miracles*. United States, Hay House.

Connect and feel secure your farmer is planting and reaping with love, if you don't get your food from a CSA - at a farmer's market you can chat with the farmers and learn about their essence and get a feel for their energy. At the farmers market, you also get to shake the hand of the person who has grown your food!

If you shop at a grocer or supermarket, consider whether they operate on the basis of conscious capitalism. Do they opt for locally grown foods as a priority? I have shopped in chain grocers that often have produce during the summer that is from local roadside stands.

Even if you have to shop at a local supermarket and have limited local produce, there are ways to improve energy and nutrients. You can buy organic seeds online and sometimes even at local grocers.

Grow your own micro-greens, mung beans, lentils and herbs on your counter top. After you soak the seeds roll them in your hands and hold them. Go ahead! Put your DNA on them!

Maybe, even consider taking a wild edibles class !

QUICK TIPS

1. Grow your own foods when possible.

2. Shop more frequently, to have fresh energy rich foods in your home.

3. Shop or pick up the items the day you will eat them.

>   *This will ensure you pick what your body is really craving!

4. Walk through the woods and check out the wild edibles in your neighborhood.

>   *Ann Wigmore actually kept herself alive by foraging for wild edibles in abandoned city lots near her home in Boston. She found hundreds of varieties of edible plant species!

SEASONAL EATING

It is a wonderful treat to eat foods from all over the world whenever we want. Consider, though, how much higher the vibrational energy of food that has been grown locally is. Even when food is grown regionally, as each day passes before consumption, the vibrational energy level decreases, nutrient levels decreases and water activity decreases! Seasonal eating will also help you to stay warm or cool down at the appropriate time of year.

LESS IS MORE

"Not too much." The majority of us simply eat too much food. The amount of food (and calories) presented on your average restaurant plate in America is astounding. Portion control, no matter what any diet plan says, is important. It's not about deprivation or starving yourself, though. It's about eating the right amount – no more, no less.

For years I thought, stuffing myself with healthy food was the answer. I thought, I could achieve optimal health by getting as much of the good stuff as possible. Eventually, I learned that even with a bounty of nutritious good to choose from, it's best to eat sparingly and choose nutrient dense foods!

At max use 5 ingredients per dish! This eases digestion and allows the opportunity to recognize and appreciate each ingredient. This will also help keep the focus on using quality ingredients. Don't eat anything with more than five ingredients or any ingredients you can't pronounce.

WATER

What to drink? Choose fresh spring water and well water when possible. At the least use filtered water in your home. Chemicals in your water will decrease the benefits to your body so it is best to consume the freshest cleanest water possible.

Check out www.findaspring.org when you have a chance !

MARIE'S TIPS

Choose:

Natural State

Local

Organic

Self-Grown

60-80% Raw

Primarily Sprouts and Greens

SUPPLEMENTS

So many people try to rectify poor food habits through supplements. Supplements are not the answer. Real whole foods nourish our bodies. Supplements can actually leach nutrients from our bodies. Also, consider the horrible energy transmitted into supplements during the manufacturing process.

True vitality is achieved through eating real foods that are grown and prepared with consciousness. Certainly there are situations when it is not possible to achieve adequate nutrients through foods alone. If you must use supplements, do so with care. Choose a reputable manufacturer who utilized real food sources!

KEEP IT SIMPLE

You don't need exotic foods, expensive shakes or supplements. Make wise intuitive choices about what foods your body needs.

And most of all **KEEP IT SIMPLE** !

Affirmations while choosing foods

Picture the food nourishing your body and soul; consider roots for grounding, leaves for respiration

Say Aloud:

This food will nourish and heal my body

I have the wisdom to choose the foods that are best for me.

I let my body guide my food choices

Chapter 3

Here, There and Everywhere
Choosing Where to Eat

We spend about a third of our lives at work. Take out the sleeping part, and most of our adult lives are actually spent working. We are meant to work. We are designed to get things done, to realize accomplishments, to – as George Bernard Shaw put it – "have it make a difference that we lived at all." Work gives meaning to our lives, and without meaning, we humans are lost. This doesn't mean we have to eat at our desks though!

The majority of us spend our workdays sitting with poor posture at our desks, glued to computer screens or telephones, lacking exposure to sunlight and fresh air.

What are the attributes of a great place to eat?

1. Quiet
2. Calming
3. Nature
4. Alone
5. Happy or Sacred place

Find somewhere beautiful and calming to eat. Somewhere that makes your feel peaceful and balanced.

What space makes you feel most balanced and centered?

For many people it is sitting outside with sunshine and a little breeze. For others it may be sitting at their grandma's dining room table.

There is no right or wrong place. It will be individual for you. Though, there is the most vibrational energy outdoors eating in nature.

One thing is certain though - **Don't eat in the car! Stop and pull over!**

You don't want to get your car messy. Plus, eating in the car will associate hunger with being in your vehicle, which can lead to overeating.

ENVIRONMENT

1. Put devices and electronics away.

2. Eat outside when possible. Sit in the grass.

3. Sit on a bench overlooking a pond.

4. The closer proximity you are to nature when you eat, the more harmonious the experience will be.

5. Wear comfortable clothing that makes you feel good.

6. Choose a calm environment.

7. Eat at home instead of a restaurant when possible.
    When dining out if the server slams the food down in from of me it affects me. This can be quite stressful to anyone's system while eating!

8. If choosing a restaurant, find one what has good ambiance or outdoor seating.

At first, you may even need to eat alone, so that you can become comfortable to resisting distraction. I have found in the past, when I am around loud or angry people, I eat more quickly and chew my food less. This leads to indigestion and inadequate absorption of nutrients. Please choose a place that works best for you.

Chapter 4

Is It Time to Eat Yet?
When To Eat

When is the best time to eat??

1. When Happy
2. When Calm
3. When Truly Hungry
4. When feeling Balanced and Supported
5. When feeling at Peace

Your mental attitude during digestion affects how the food will be assimilated and utilized.

Your frame of mind and thoughts for several hours after eating matter!

Don't eat when tired. Rest first.

Gratitude

While eating say: THANK YOU for your plates, bowl, cup, fork, napkins and table. Focus on the items supporting the food as well as the food itself.

When To Eat

1. The daily detoxification process goes from 11pm to 11am. Do not eat during this time, unless advised by to your doctor that it is medically necessary.

2. Sun guided eating. The digestive enzymes in our bodies are most active when the sun is highest in the sky. This is why it makes sense to eat your biggest meal of the day around midday.

3. Give food optimal time to digest. It takes to 1.5 hours for food to digest. **Do not plan meetings or stressful events immediately after eating. Optimally go for a minimum of a 10 minutes walk after eating. 30 minutes if possible**.

4. Before making food for yourself or consuming it ask yourself - if I truly completed loved and accepted myself would I eat this now?

THOUGHTS TO CONSIDER
BEFORE EATING

Cravings aren't actually hunger.

Did you know ice cream can actually be a desire for more love and hugs?

Do you really need more love in your life? Many emotions may be actually be mistaken for hunger.

What time of the day do you feel most relaxed? This is the best time to eat your main meal. Optimally, it is best to eat your main meal of the day when the sun is highest in the sky because this is the time the enzymes in our stomach is most active. Eating at this time will not be optimal for you if midday is an especially stressful time for you.

It is also thought that good and bad microbes play a part in our mood. Stress kills good microbe and calm supports the growth of healthy microbes. When we are stressed our good microbes are reduced. **Eating while stressed causes even more stress out our body and spirit. This is why it's important to eat while calm.**

Although, it's very important to have family dinners to connect and bond. This could be a very stressful time for you. It is more important to care for yourself than to just ingest good because you are at a dinner table. You can still sit with your family and sip water or tea so that you can partake in the conversation without harming your body. If necessary, you can always make a plate and wrap it to eat later when you are alone and feeling calm.

If your family is particularly demanding about consuming meals together, opt mitigate conflict. Make a plate of food and leave it in front of you while others eat. They will be so busy tending to their own plates that they won't notice that you aren't eating. Then, just save the plate for later when you are feeling relaxed and truly hungry.

It may not be ideal to tell family members that you feel to stressed to eat around them. Just opt for the path of least resistance and say you aren't hungry at that time.

Eating while rushing

So many times, I felt I was doing myself a favor by eating the car. I thought, that way, I could be more productive and get as much done possible in one day. I didn't realize that I was robbing myself the enjoyment of eating. Really smelling and tasting it. Savoring the texture. I was really just hampering my body's digestion. When your eyes are focused on the road, your focus is on driving and getting to your destination; your body's primary intention is not on digestion. Thus, the food goes down your throat and sits there like a **LUMP** in your stomach because your body is busy concentrating on something else.

So, you're not doing yourself a favor by eating while you're driving. You're actually putting more stress on your body. If you really feel incredibly hungry and need to drive somewhere, then it's time to make a choice. Can you take that 5 or 10 minutes that you need to have a little snack? It takes just a couple minutes to eat celery or an apple. Or is it best for you to get to make it to your destination, then eat?

Recently, I ate a handful of organic locally grown celery while driving. I have to say, that the first couple pieces of celery were so sweet and delicious. Yet, the rest was horrible! It was because I was focused on getting to my destination on time. There was no flavor, vitality or energy. It just shows that you can eat food that is free of pesticides and a solid healthy choice but if you are in an environment that's not nourishing, the poor energy is going to transfer.

Did you know that what you think, feel and believe can affect your microbiology? Physical and emotional stress will decrease the population of good bugs and increase the population of bad bugs in your body. Healthy microbiology is dependent on the foods we eat and our microbiology affects our brain.

So, it's not just a matter of choosing what simply tastes good. Increasing the amount of good bugs in our system is also very calming and helps mitigate stress. Eating the right foods now will in turn help you make better choices it the future because good bugs improve memory, mood and focus function.

FAT AND STRESS

Are you aware that the fat on your body is actually saving your life and is a protective mechanism? Our body deposits the fat so that our systems don't get too acidic, which would be very hazardous to our health. So, your fat has actually been saving you all these years! You should consider gratitude to your fat for saving your life.

Want to remove fat and stop depositing more? **Calm down. Relax. Feel.** This will alkalize your body.

72

Our bodies are not designed to thrive on long-term constant stress. Enjoying a low stress, high vibrational life is the to longevity and happiness.

Looking back, I've wasted so many meals being anxious. So much money on the "right" foods, not realizing my mindset and emotion at the time of eating was reeling havoc on my body. I thought, how could my hair being falling out, my stomach be in pain and to feel so lethargic when I was putting such high quality food in body?

The answer is that I was putting toxic emotions and energy into my body. Creating building blocks full of holes and negative energy.

Our genes used to be considered fixed. It was thought that they controlled all aspects of our physical body and, perhaps, even behavior characteristics.

New research indicates that how you think, feel, speak and act actually affects our genomes.

Chapter 5
Putting Yourself Into Your Food
How to Prepare Foods

Did you know that electromagnetic power of the heart is 5,000 times stronger than that of the brain?

Do you think you are doing yourself or your family any good if you are preparing a meal while full of anxiety thinking about a stressful day a work?

Do you think you are nourishing your family, if you are full of anger and rage?

Preparing or Cooking is fun and grounding!

Putting in:
1. Love
2. Peace
3. Energy

Do you think you are doing yourself or your family any good if you are preparing a meal while full of anxiety thinking about a stressful day a work?
Do you think you are nourishing your family, if you are full of anger and rage?

PREPARATION

Picture your family or friends enjoying the meal. Picture yourself smiling and enjoying the meal. I suggest you concentrate on your love of your children while preparing a meal.

Preparing a meal for your spouse or significant other? Focus on your admiration and respect for that person.

Prepare food while calm. As you are cutting and chopping, do so with care. Wash each vegetable and piece of fruit with love and intention. Selection the utensils and plates with care.

Focus on loving intentions. Open your heart. Think and concentrate on those that you are making the food for and your love for them. Think about how much they mean to you and how much you want them to be healthy and happy. Nourish them with your intentions.

If you are making food for yourself, then concentrate on your love for yourself. Kneed the food thoroughly using your hands.

Put your heart into what you are making. Don't answer the phone or watch TV while preparing food. Let all your feelings and emotions will go into the food you are preparing.

If you don't like or trust someone don't let them make food you! Especially, if you feel they don't have your best intentions in mind.

Those negative emotions will transfer to the food and will also tell your body to slow down digestion because it is fearful of the bad intention from the preparer. Your body does not want to be poisoned physically or emotionally.

SCHOOL LUNCHES

Think about how much you love your child and wish them well. While making lunch for your child, think, "I love you".

While cutting the apples and cucumber send the thought this thought to them "you will have an amazing day. I am so blessed to love and guide you. I am so blessed to be your parent. Say thank you for the gift of being able to care for your child.

Also, promote your child making their own lunch with your assistance so they can put their own "secret ingredient" into the food.

INTENTIONS

In his book *Integrative Nutrition*, Joshua Rosenthal discusses a spiritual guide who knew when his students had been hurried, stressed or anxious while preparing a meal, just by eating the food. This demonstrates a recognizable conveyance of energy. Being able to recognize energy at this level can take years of practice but begin simply by concentrating on your intentions.

Often times, in the past, I found my mind wandering while preparing meals. Straying to: Anxiety, Fear, Regret and Worry. Unfortunately, all these thoughts will transfer to the food.

When you are at home preparing foods, earthing can provide the grounding necessary to feel balance and centered. If possible, stand outside in the grass at a picnic table while you prepare a fresh salad. Taking in the sights, sounds and feel of nature will help you convey love and gratitude while you prepare the meal!

While setting the table, you can also convey energy by thinking "I love you" and directing to yourself and your family.

Affirmation to focus on while preparing foods

I love myself

I am safe

I am perfect

I am happy

I am loving

I am strong

I am whole

I am loving

I am harmonious

"The only emotion with higher vibrational energy than love is gratitude" –Massaru Emoto

TRANSFERRING YOUR ENERGY

Our vibrations transfer to our food. It is vital to eat foods with the highest vibrational energy.

In order to convey the maximum energy, I suggest you use stoneware, wood, glass or ceramic. Artificial materials such a plastics may hinder the transfer of positive energy.

Be mindful of forgiveness. Forgive yourself and forgive others. You cannot move on from where you are now without letting go of the past. Without it, we would not be where we are now. So, show gratitude for the road you have traveled and where it has gotten you. To erase the past would to change where you are now.

Even the act of peeling an orange can be an act of love. Think. Reflect. Focus. Be mindful. Think about how much you love the person you are preparing the food for whether it be a family member, friend or yourself.

While making lunch for your child, think, "I love you". While cutting the apples and cucumber, send this thought to them, "you will have an amazing day. I am so blessed to love and guide you. I am so blessed to be your parent." Also, say thank you for the gift of being able to care for your child.

Before preparing food for your family, ask yourself: if I truly loved them would I make, bake, prepare or buy this?

Before making food for yourself or consuming it ask yourself - if I truly completed loved and accepted myself would I eat this? Would I make this for myself?

Sometimes, when other people prepare for me, the same food I normally love and enjoy, I feel horrible. It is because their energy is passed to me through the food. This is why it is best to make your own food and even grow your own food when possible; even if you can only grow countertop sprouts and micro greens.

FENG SHUI

Make the food appealing to the eye. This sense is very important and affects our perception of the food. You may even want to consider the room Feng Shui while you eat. Are things cluttered or neat? Body Feng Shui: relax, breathe deep and wear loose fitting clothes while eating.

If you are mad at yourself or your family members don't cook!

Calm down. Relax. Convey positive energy.

ADDITIONAL AFFIRMATIONS WHILE PREPARING FOOD

I love and approve of myself.

It is safe for me to care for myself.

There is time and space for everything I need to do.

It is my birthright to live fully and freely.

I am worth loving.

I now choose to live life fully.

Chapter 6
Slow Down Cowboy!
The Art of Eating

What you think, say and do today affects your genetic future. We can smell trillions of different scents. Just the scent of food can carry emotionally charged feelings and memories. This can trigger a cascade of memories and an ingrained psychological response. It can even determine whether or not you like the food, independent of the actual taste.

Appreciate the current moment for what it is. Be present in your own life.

Consider:

1. Slowing Down
2. Feeling Gratitude
3. Using Your Hands
4. Feeling Your Connection To Others

Consider your food a gift that we must treat as such. The energy of the sun has gone into the leaves of plants and when we eat those plants we are able to heal ourselves.

Eat with people you love and feel at ease with. Surround yourself with love and light.

Drink Minimal liquids while eating. Always have a side of cucumbers on your plate. They will act as your water but not hamper digestion.

Hurry is poison!!!!

Chew. Chew. Chew. Slowly…..

Go beyond the physical makeup of your food and infuse positive emotional charge. This is why is so important to make your food appealing to the eye.

Even reading while eating hampers digestion. Not focusing on the food distracts our body and slows digestion. When eating a mantra such as "my body digests this food with ease and absorbs nutrients readily" may be useful.

At maximum use 5 ingredients per dish. This eases digestion and allows the opportunity to recognize and appreciate each ingredient. This will also help keep the focus on using quality ingredients.

Consider closing your eye while chewing and swallowing. When our eyes are closed our other senses are heightened. Also, before you begin eating-close your eyes inhale deeply and truly smell the food. Closing your eyes will increase flavor.

Put your fork down in between bites and truly focus on what you are eating!

Music also affects flavor. Silence amplifies flavors. Slow music can help dictate pace.

EVERYDAY PRACTICE

Breathe. You may not be able to embody all these techniques every minute of every day. Be kind to yourself. Start with one step at a time. Perhaps, choosing or growing your foods with care. Put love into the process of bringing foods into your life. Beverages matter too. Try some fresh lemonade that you have juiced with your own hands and sweetened with fresh pressed stevia. Enjoy feeling the love and energy you have put into making yourself such a delicious refreshing beverage.

Always eat with your hands when possible or hygienic. **Be sure to wash your hands before eating**

Also consider mono meals as a practice to enhance perception of flavor, smell and texture.

Feng Shui your plate and environment so you feel calm as well as grounded.

CHEW. CHEW. CHEW.

In order to fully release the nutrients and maximize the full potential of your food, you must chew is thoroughly. The experts say you should drink your food and chew your beverages! The chewing action stimulates the gastric juices in our stomach aiding in proper digestion.

WHILE EATING

Think about the taste

* Hold the Food in your mouth*

* Experience gratitude*

Feel the Food nourishing your body

Eat meals with a combination of sensations: crunchy, soft, warming and cooling sensations

ADDITIONAL TIPS

Let veggies sit out at room temperature before eating. Optimally, pluck from your garden or buy just before eating then prepare without refrigerating.

Consider closing your eye while chewing and swallowing. When our eyes are closed our other senses are heightened. Before you begin eating-close your eyes inhale deeply and truly smell the food.

FOCUS

Give yourself plenty of time to eat. You don't want to feel rushed.

Consider whether music and your surrounding are a hindrance or beneficial.

No phones or tablets while eating.

Eat from plates you really like. Use beautiful cups and glasses. Get dressed up and wear your best clothes.

Be mindful of forgiveness. Forgiveness. Forgive yourself and forgive others. You cannot move on from where you are now without letting go of the past. Without it, we would not be where we are now. So, show gratitude for the road you have traveled and where it has gotten you. **To erase the past would to change where you are now.**

Consider blessing your food at the start of a meal by offering thanks and truly feeling gratitude for what you are about to receive. I also suggest that you focus on your love of yourself and your aim to nourish your body through the food you are consuming. Additionally, ending a meal with gratitude re-centers us and aids in digestion.

Consider how admonishing yourself for eating fried food or ice cream may actually hamper your digestion and make things tougher on your body.

Take your shoes off.

Wear comfortable clothing. (Organic natural fibers if possible)

Give plenty of time before hand to be calm and relax before eating. 30 minutes of calming is ideal. Take a walk, if possible. Even just a few minutes help clam and center the mind and body. Walking will also stimulate the digestive system.

1.5 hours necessary for digestion. Walk after eating for 15 - 30 minutes.

Focus on belly breathing while eating and digesting. Proper posture while eating will enhance digestion and assimilation of nutrients. Notice whether you typically eat hunched over and how it makes you feel.

Close your eyes. Smell the food and enjoy the aroma. Inhales. Feel the texture. Savor the taste.

While chewing repeat these thoughts: I Love Myself. I am safe. Thank you. I am nourished. I am safe.

FOOD FOR THOUGHT

While eating consider gratitude to the people who grew your food, transported it and prepared it and cooked it.

Perception is everything. A situation that is stressful to you may be calming to someone else. Be patient with others. Yet, you must still consider your own person needs above others when it comes to nourishing your body.

Always leave the table a little hungry. Aim for 3/4 full.

Taking time and truly relaxing is actually more important that what and when you eat. According to Ayurveda - the key to healthy eating is becoming aware of what we are eating through our senses.

Mindset or emotional state at the time of eating will emotionally charge the food. If you are relaxed and calm the food will be positively charged.

If you are stressed, the food will be charged will hurry and stress. If you are upset or depressed the food will be negatively charged. The charge will in turn actually affect the "nutrient essence" of the food.

Digestion starts the moment we sense the presence of food. Our mouths begin to water. Our stomach begins to rumble.

The sight, smell, taste, touch and sound of food emotionally charges it with positive or negative vibrational energy. In Sanskrit the words for emotion and taste are the same.

In some countries it is customary to eat with your fingers. It is thought that each finger represents in of the five senses.

This way of eating with the fingers allows all the senses to be stimulated and become part of the process of eating.

The food we eat is the foundation for our bodies and each cell is emotional charged based on the experience of the senses at the time of eating.

Try to take only small sips of water while eating. Allow your body to digest at it's full potential.

Some days you may be able to embody all the steps. Other days, none at all. Be kind to yourself. Each moment and each minute is new. Just because you chose or ate your lunch hastily doesn't mean that the intention for the day is ruined. BREATHE. Continue from that moment forward with intention and love.

AFFIRMATIONS WHILE EATING

The world is safe and friendly.

I am at peace with life.

I love and approve of myself,

I trust the process of life.

I am safe.

Life agrees with me.

I assimilate the new every moment of every day. All is well.

There is time and space for everything I need to do.

I now choose to live life fully.

Remember eating starts with the eyes:

Display fresh fruits and vegetables on countertops in wooden and ceramic bowls so start the process of your body craving healthful foods.

Store foods in clear glass containers. Arrange them in a visually appealing way.

Your refrigerator should be a display of beauty not just functionality. Arrange healthy food in a way that appeals to the eye.

Buy foods of different shapes, sizes and colors. Use a mandolin or spiralizer to make various shapes and size snacks. Mix and match textures.

Chapter 7
Stop Right There!
When Not To Eat

WHEN SHOULDN'T YOU EAT?

If you are feeling:
1. Emotional
2. Hurried
3. In a Hectic environment
4. Not truly hungry

Our energy goes right into our food!

When we are feeling anxious or upset, it is best not to consume anything until we are centered and balanced again. Our digestion is severely hampered when we are upset, angry, stressed.

Learn and know how to stop eating. Understand what being full feels like. Anger can be mistaken for hunger. Lighter foods won't leave you with that same lump in your gut feeling.

Emotions can often times be mistaken as hunger. Most often people mistake anger for hunger, though some do mistake happiness for hunger.

Eating this way will make you feel lighter. It is important to get used to this feeling and not mistake it for hunger. Traditional eating can cause a lump in our stomachs, which is a sign of overeating not fullness.

If you don't like or trust someone don't let them make food you. This is also true if you feel they don't have your best intentions in mind. Those negative emotions will transfer to the food and will also tell your body to slow down digestion because it is fearful of the negative energy from the preparer.

Likewise, if you are mad at someone - do make food for him or her! You will harm them, even though it is not apparent physically.

Always leave the table a little hungry. Aim for 3/4 full.

Mindset or emotional state at the time of eating will emotionally charge the food. If you are relaxed and calm the food will be positively charged. If you are stressed, the food will be charged will hurry and stress.

If you are upset or depressed the food will be negatively charged. The charge can actually affect the "nutrient essence" of the food.

Depression. If you are feeling down, consider options to improve your mood and feelings. Volunteer. Annonymously do something nice for another feeling - helping other can dramatically change our sense of well-being within minutes.

If you need to forgive, it may be best to tackle this before gobbling down food. Forgiveness could be holding you back.

Affirmations for forgiveness:

I easily release that which I no longer need. The past is over, and I am free.

Forgiveness doesn't hurt the other person it hurts you. It makes you stressed. It affects your life. By holding onto to the past, it difficult to move forward into the future and the peace you are meant to have.

For years I had not forgiven my mother for not being there for me physically and emotionally. When I came to peace and acceptance of her as she is, not how I wished she was, my life changed dramatically.

When you aren't up to eating consider these options instead or do these, then see if you feel well enough to eat:

Laugh for 10 minutes each day. Improves immune system. Reduces stress. Improves overall happiness.

Find a Laughter Yoga group.

Go to comedy clubs.

Watch comedy clips online.

Watch funny movies.

Laugh with friends.

If you have determined that it is not the best time to eat:

1. Go for a walk outside barefoot
2. Breath in fresh air and practice belly breathing
3. Go outside and feel sunshine on your face
4. Consider everything you are grateful for
5. Ask yourself power questions and consider your accomplishments in life.

When dining out it can be stressful for your body Stressful. Even if you are at a restaurant you can choose not to eat if you become stressed. Breath deep, wait until you feel calm and centered. If that does not happen - ask to have the food boxed and bring it home. **You must never feel forced to EAT!**

AFFIRMATIONS

If you are not feeling centered and calm enough to eat but are truly hungry, these affirmations may help:

The world is safe and friendly.

I am safe.

I am at peace with life.

I love and approve of myself,

I trust the process of life.

I am safe.

I easily release that which I no longer need.

The past is over, and I am free.

Affirmations for excessive appetite

I am safe.

It is safe to feel.

My feelings are normal and acceptable.

Affirmations for loss of appetite

I love and approve of myself.

I am safe.

Life is safe and joyous.

Chapter 8
Looking Back
After Eating

Did you know that your mental attitude during digestion affects how the food will be assimilated and utilized?

1. Consider how you feel physically - did you eat too much?
2. Gratitude - are you thankful for what it took to grow, prepare, raise you r food?
3. Digestion - walk after eating
4. How do you feel emotionally? Did the food quench an emotion or do you feel light yet nourished?
5. What is your level of awareness?

Are you cold? Drowsy? Lethargic? Achy? Bloats?

Consider food combining and possible food allergies.

Did you eat at a bad time?

Were you focusing? Or distracted while

eating?

Were you feeling gratitude or guilt while eating?

Were you arguing or discussing a heated topic while eating?

What can you do to improve the experience next time?

The secret ingredient is not only about bringing food and drink into our lives and bodies with love but also to release with love. Optional digestion requires proper food combining, walking, probiotics and water in our systems. And of course, the ability to let go of the past and make way for the future.

As important as it us for us to make healthy food choices and to put love into our food, it is important to be aware that we not judge others who do not do this. If someone is not at the same place in their journey as you, lead by examples and they will catch on little by little. Forcing something upon another will not yield positive results.

We all get to where we need to go in our own time. Don't avoid others just because you don't approve if their food choices or way of eating. This can be isolating and just as detrimental as not using the secret ingredient. Be around others spread your light.

Relate to people without judgment. Do not preach. Let others do as they wish. Then when you least expect it the will ask about what they have noticed you doing. Even then it is important to explain what you do and tell them what they should be doing.

Remember that you love others regardless of how they look, what they eat or what choices they make in life. What other people do is not your business. Your only business is to love them unconditionally.

If being around someone else actively harms your health, then it is your right to stay away from him or her and silently wish then well as they continue on their journey.

AFFIRMATIONS AFTER EATING

Letting go is easy

I freely and easily release the old and joyously welcome the new.

I easily release that which I no longer need.

The past is over, and I am free.

I digest and assimilate all new experiences peacefully and joyously.

Chapter 9
Special Considerations

Too much of a good thing is still bad. Eating very healthy but eating too much was a common theme for me in the past.

Overeating harms the body and slows down healing. Listen to your body. Are you truly hungry? Do you need a hug? Let your body take a break. It is not necessary to eat 3 meals a day or even eat everyday. Let your body and intuition be your guide.

My daughter is a great example, some days she eats 5 meals. Other days, she just nibble a few apples, here and there. Let your body tell you what it needs. Often times it turns out when my daughter is eating much more than usual that she has grown an inch or two taller. Our bodies are intuitively intelligent.

Also, consider mono meals as a practice to enhance perception of flavor, smell and texture.

At max use 5 ingredients per dish. This eases digestion and allows the opportunity the recognize and appreciate each ingredient. This will also help keep the focus on using quality ingredients.

When you need whimsy in your life use the spiral user. Feeling serious - julienne. Circle cut veggies for kids. Want to feel powerful? Cut your carrots into lightening bolts. When you are looking for variety in your life, mix textures and consume foods with vibrant colors

In life, we are getting bit all the time. It's not the bite that kills us, it's the venom circulating in our system if we don't release it. Better yet, we can transmute what was once toxic and turn it into medicine.

What you think, say and do today affects your genetic future.

Take time and care to make something special for a friend who is sad or upset. Transfer your love and positive energy to them with the food you make. Take great care in electing the ingredients. Put energy and intention into the meal as you prepare it. Present the food in a beautiful manner.

What am I telling you? Money and stature do not make a difference in your health. Love does. Love yourself enough to slow down and feel gratitude for yourself, your family and the offerings before you.

If you are a busy person, what you can do right now to improve the absorption of nutrients and ENERGY is to slow down! Live with gratitude.

Wake up in the morning and start your day with gratitude. List 100 things, people and events you are truly grateful for.

Try Tony Robbins' Power Questions to get you in a mindset of gratitude!

What if you are feeling stressed that you have to go buy something for dinner for your family because what you have on hand isn't good enough? Slow down. Breathe. Give gratitude for all the food already in your house, then use your love to come up with a creative idea for using the items you already have. Think to yourself, "wow, I sure am lucky to have all these options at my fingertips" Putting energy, love and creativity into those items is what will make them even more special.... plus you won't have to "waste" extra time going to the store.

Many of the great geniuses of their time realized that raw fruits, veggies, nuts and seeds naturally have higher vibrational energy. That is a great starting point, but you can put even more energy into those foods with your LOVE.

Are you having trouble slowing down? As Bruce Lipton demonstrated to us in his book *The Biology of Belief,* environment is everything.

So, if you need a hand, take a look at your environment. Is your home cluttered? Do you feel stressed when you look around? Disorganized? Rushed? Like you are drowning?

Trying to center yourself and prepare food in that environment will be a tough task unless you have horse blinders on. So, the first step in putting energy into your food may actually be tidying up your home and maybe even financial affairs. Try making a list of dinners for the week. You don't have to follow it 100% and you can even flip menus items from different days but just having the tentative dinner plan for the week up on the refrigerator will be a breathe of fresh air.... and certainly something to be grateful for.

Another action that will advance you toward putting more of the secret ingredient into your life is having a weekly house cleaning list or chore list. I have a chart that I print out each week, which I lovingly call "the clean house project". The chart designates daily chores and day specific chores. Then when the chores get done. The person who completed the item initials that block. This not only gives a sense of peace knowing when a certain task is supposed to be done but also gives pride and ownership to the person who completes the item.

Whether you do all the cleaning yourself or outsource, this chart is still very useful. I, for instance, have determined after years being assigned to laundry as a child, that I would rather bring clothes to the laundry center to have someone else wash and fold them. The sense of peace, ease and relief I get from paying a meager amount of money to have someone else fold my laundry is amazing. Even though this task is outsourced - I have this item designated on my "clean house" calendar - Tuesday designated as my "drop off laundry day" and wed as the pick up day. So, even if you pay a house cleaner, lawn mower, laundry person, and dry cleaner - the day for this should be designated on your project clean house calendar.

Another very important way to be able to "activate" the secret ingredient in your life is by bringing ease into your financial life. The simplest way to start with this is to begin saving a small amount each week. Determine how much you can afford to put aside and designate an amount to automatically transfer to your savings each week. Just the act of beginning to save will reduce stress and bring more gratitude into your life.

The next step would be to start tracking your expenditures and repeating expenses. Get a clear idea of how much you spend each month, if you don't already know. Ultimately, then you should be able to create a budget. Most people don't follow a budget but there is ease in knowing you have one.

Another great step in reducing stress is to reduce expenses. Determine expenditures you can cut back on. Having a lower base of expenses will also ease the burden.

Chapter 10

Your Thoughts Are Food

We create our future. We control our genes and direct which characteristics/traits turn on and off through our words, thoughts and actions.

If you eat food full of stress and hurry not only will you affect your cells negatively but it will also affect your food. With high stress energy food vibrating in your body it can't be easy to be calm and relaxed. Direct your own biology. Create your own life and live it fully.

This makes me think of a very compelling story that I remember reading in Tony Robbins' *Classic Awaken the Power Within*. He tells of a man who was imprisoned, served dirty water and moldy bread. Yet, he thrived and made it through 7 years as a POW! This shows, it's all about your energy, intention and focus. This man focused on the food nourishing and sustaining him; the result was undeniable.

Your thoughts are food. This is why there are people who can enjoy heavy fatty foods and not see changes to their waistline. They consume foods prepared by family members in a loving environment and feel the nourishment and energy in the food.

There are only two states of being in life. LOVE and FEAR. Choose LOVE.

Chapter 11
Putting It All Together

7 Steps to transform your food and your life

Actions consistent with the secret ingredient

1. Aim to consume 60-80% of your foods as raw fruits vegetables, nuts and seeds to obtain maximum vitality from your food.

2. When preparing foods focus on love and intention.

3. Choose to eat away from distractions such as TV, phone, and loud music, hectic environments

4. Offer gratitude for your food at the beginning and end of your meal.

5. While eating focus on the taste, color, texture and sensation of the food. Consider how you are nourishing your body.

6. Eat with you hands when possible. Make eating a tactile experience and energy transfer readily available.

7. CHEW. Chew. Chew.

Most importantly, you don't need special foods, expensive shakes, supplements or anything. You just need your own mind and thoughts. Perception dictates behavior. - Put this sentiment at the beginning of the book and again at the end.

Affirmations are our best friend. Although, I have offered affirmations for all situations most simply remember - I love and approve of myself. I am safe. All is well.

You are extraordinary, powerful and unstoppable. Everything takes time. Practice one transforming step at a time. Practice each step for three weeks before moving on to the next. It takes 21 days to fully create a habit.

Help mentor others to love themselves more.

Embrace your shadow.

"There would not be light without darkness" - Deepak Choprah.

We all have light and dark. Embrace it.

Breathe.

You may not be able to embody all these techniques every minute of every day. Be kind to yourself. Start with one step at a time. Perhaps, choosing or growing your foods with care.

Put love into the process of bringing foods into your life. Beverages matter too. Focus on love and positive intention as you refresh yourself with liquid nourishment as well.

When we started this journey, I referred to the secret ingredient as something you could add or put in and you may have thought of the secret ingredients something outside yourself.

The reality is that the secret ingredient is about putting yourself, your soul and your energy into your food and your life.

You are the LOVE.

The answer has always been inside you.

And is you.

Thus, the answer to "What is the Secret Ingredient?"

"I AM" "YOU ARE" "WE ARE"

Chapter 12

Community

You want to know what made Weight Watchers and Jenny Craig such popular weight loss programs? It wasn't the packaged foods or the point system.

It was the support.

It was the fact that people who wanted to lose weight didn't feel so isolated. They felt – and continue to feel – like they have a group of people who can empathize with their struggles and give them encouragement when they feel like they can't hang on.

No one has ever achieved optimum health all alone. Part of the reason is that isolation itself is an unhealthy habit… again, if taken to excess.

We are a social species, and we need others around us… not just for social reasons, work reasons, and family reasons. We need others around us for support, community, guidance, and accountability.

We live in a society where potential sabotage lurks around every corner. It lurks in the form of processed foods designed to steal from our taste buds the joy of eating real foods. It lurks in the confusing and untrue health claims made on the outside of packaged foods.

It lurks in the form of sedentary jobs, followed by evenings spent in front of the television and other mindless forms of entertainment that keep us from getting up and moving to entertain ourselves.

And it lurks in social gatherings, restaurants, and the media.

Not only does getting healthy seem like too much work, but also it's overwhelming just thinking about where to begin, and how to sustain the effort.

Support in the form of a group of people who have the same goals can be very valuable. But personal, one-on-one support and guidance from a trained professional can also be just what you need.

Imagine having someone with specialized knowledge and the ability to apply it directly to you, dedicated to personally helping you wade through all the unique factors that conspire to keep you unhealthy!

If, like many people, you find going it alone to be too difficult, there are people and places you can turn to for support. Enlist a friend, join a Meetup group or get help from a professional!

This will help you gain clarity about your current situation from the very start. You'll begin to understand the factors that are getting in your way, and you'll see the path to health and wellness beyond what you imagined.

Move Past Obstacles

It can also be helpful to break down and address the three primary obstacles to making lasting changes:

1.   It's too hard to make all these changes at once.

It IS hard to make too many changes at once. And for most people, such attempts fail. That's why we don't make all the changes at once. The body is very resilient and responds well to even the smallest changes intended to yield improvements. Improvements you'll feel empowered to maintain and improve upon - for the rest of your life. Remember, it's not a race to "get there" as fast as you can. The point is to make lasting changes that will add years to your life and life to your years.

2.   It's too confusing to know exactly what to do.

The confusion in the world of food and nutrition these days is crazy. Take time to learn about how to benefit from nutrient density, healthy cooking techniques, what food labels and ingredients really mean, how and where to shop.

Custom tailor a plan that works for your body and in your life. Because remember, one size DOES NOT fit all. A book or a program can get you started in the right direction. But it takes time, patience, and support to get where you ultimately need to go.

Take Action !

Awareness
Use a journal or smartphone app to track what you eat and how you feel. Awareness is the first step toward healthy living.

Upgrade Your Foods
Get lots of greens, lots of vegetables and plenty of water.

Prepare For Success
Plan ahead. Pack and keep these handy at work and on the road: nuts, veggies, fruit and whole food bars.

Balance Your Circle of Life
Fill yourself up with healthy relationships, thoughtful spirituality, meaningful work and energizing physical activity.

Get A Buddy
No one has ever achieved optimum health alone. We need each other for support, guidance, community and accountability.

Lifestyle Balance

The food we eat is foundational. It really can change everything – especially the way we feel, both physically and mentally. Of course, these good feelings can also lead to many other areas of improvement in our lives. And they often do. Recent studies have even shown that longevity might actually have more to do with these other areas in our lives than with the food we eat.

It all goes together. If you start eating well, you give yourself the best possible foundation for a well-functioning machine (your body) that can handle the particulars of all the other truly more important aspects of your life.

These are strange times we live in. On the one hand, we are living on average almost twice as long as our ancestors lived a hundred years ago. Twice as long! That's an amazing leap in life expectancy.

We certainly do owe a lot of that to science and modern medicine, to the eradication of many diseases, and to surgical procedures and pharmaceuticals that allow us to confront mortal dangers in ways unthinkable throughout most of human history.

And yet, most of us spend the last few years of our longer lives battling diseases that we brought on ourselves - diseases that were unheard of in generations past. Heart disease is the number one killer, followed closely by cancer and strokes come in at number three. We blindly accept these conditions as a normal part of growing older, because "we're all going to die from something."

I'm not so sure this is "living" longer. It's existing, but is it truly living? And death from "natural causes" is a very rare cause of death these days indeed.

It's no surprise, though, that we resign ourselves to that sort of death. It's a logical end to the kind of lives so many of us lead - more of an 'existence' for the sake of surviving, not thriving.

We run from one moment to the next, satisfying needs and wants based on the premise of immediate gratification, without taking much time to look at the whole picture in our lives.

We rush out the door to work in the morning, plow through the stresses of the tasks before us in fear of losing our jobs because we have bills to pay, not because the work has any deeper meaning for us.

We grab the food that's most convenient and tastes good to our dulled taste buds, not the foods our bodies need to thrive. We rarely sit down to eat, and when we do, we're often alone, in front of the television or computer, mindless images and entertainment taking up valuable space in our brains.

We sit far more often than we stand, drive when we could walk, take elevators when the stairs are right there. We spend more time texting than talking, taking our spouses for granted and forgetting to participate in our children's growth to adulthood.

How many of us truly take the time to meditate, to think, to pray, to be?

We are each given one precious life. And if we're really going to live it, we need to have a holistic approach to it. Health and happiness don't just happen. We must look at all aspects of our lives.

Eating well is critically important, but it alone cannot fill our souls.

Encouragement

The best action you can take is to set an example by maximizing your own health. When you upgrade your life, your family and friends will see the changes. They may not say anything immediately nor will they adopt any changes for quite some time. Rest assured, though, they are on notice. Soon, they will see improvements in your health and energy. Then, they will want the same for themselves!

I hope this book has helped you make some simple but significant changes in your health already. There isn't a one size fits all solution to our health, but it's an ironic truth that replacing technology, efficiency and convenience with nourishment, authenticity, and joy yields the most amazing results.

It's by simplifying, not complicating, our approach to life that we can lead a richer and fuller one.

I wish you all the best!

About The Author

Marie Ann Mosher is an Academy of Sports Medicine Certified Personal Trainer and Internationally Certified Integrative Health Coach. She is graduate of the University of Connecticut, where she studied Nutritional Science as well as Occupational Health and Safety. Marie is also a graduate of the Institute for Integrative Nutrition in New York City, where she studied more than one hundred dietary theories and a variety of practical lifestyle teaching methods with some of the world's top health and wellness experts. She's written many books including Beyond Food, The Secret Ingredient, Secret Weight Loss Hacks and the Biohacker Secrets Series. Marie also hosts the Secret Weight Loss Hacks Free Facebook support community. You can join here - https://www.facebook.com/groups/secretweightlosshacks/

Marie previously collaborated with food industry leaders to create and market healthier foods. She has developed several products currently in Supermarkets across the country including Whole Foods and previously owned an Organic Raw Foods Cafe. Please visit **www.marieannmosher.com** for more inspiration and free recipes.

Invite Marie to Speak to Your Group or Organization

Marie is an inspiring and dynamic professional speaker. Her audiences include groups and organizations of every size and type.

Topic Specialties:

Self Care Mastery
Stress Management
Homes Designed for Health
Healthy Business Strategies
Healing through Primary Food
Lifestyle Balance

For more information go to
www.marieannmosher.com

Connect with Marie

www.marieannmosher.com

www.amazon.com/author/marieannmosher

www.facebook.com/marieAnnmosher

www.facebook.com/rawathlete

www.twitter.com/marieannmosher

www.linkedin.com/in/mariemosher

www.instagram.com/marieannmosher